Male Body Positive

JOSH J JONES

Copyright © 2024 by Josh J Jones
All rights reserved.
No portion of this book may be reproduced in any form without written permission from the publisher or author, except as permitted by U.S. copyright law.

"It was men who stopped slavery. It was men who ran up the stairs in the Twin Towers to rescue people. It was men who gave up their seats on the lifeboats of the Titanic. Men are made to take risks and live passionately on behalf of others." John Eldredge

For al the men who ever felt less

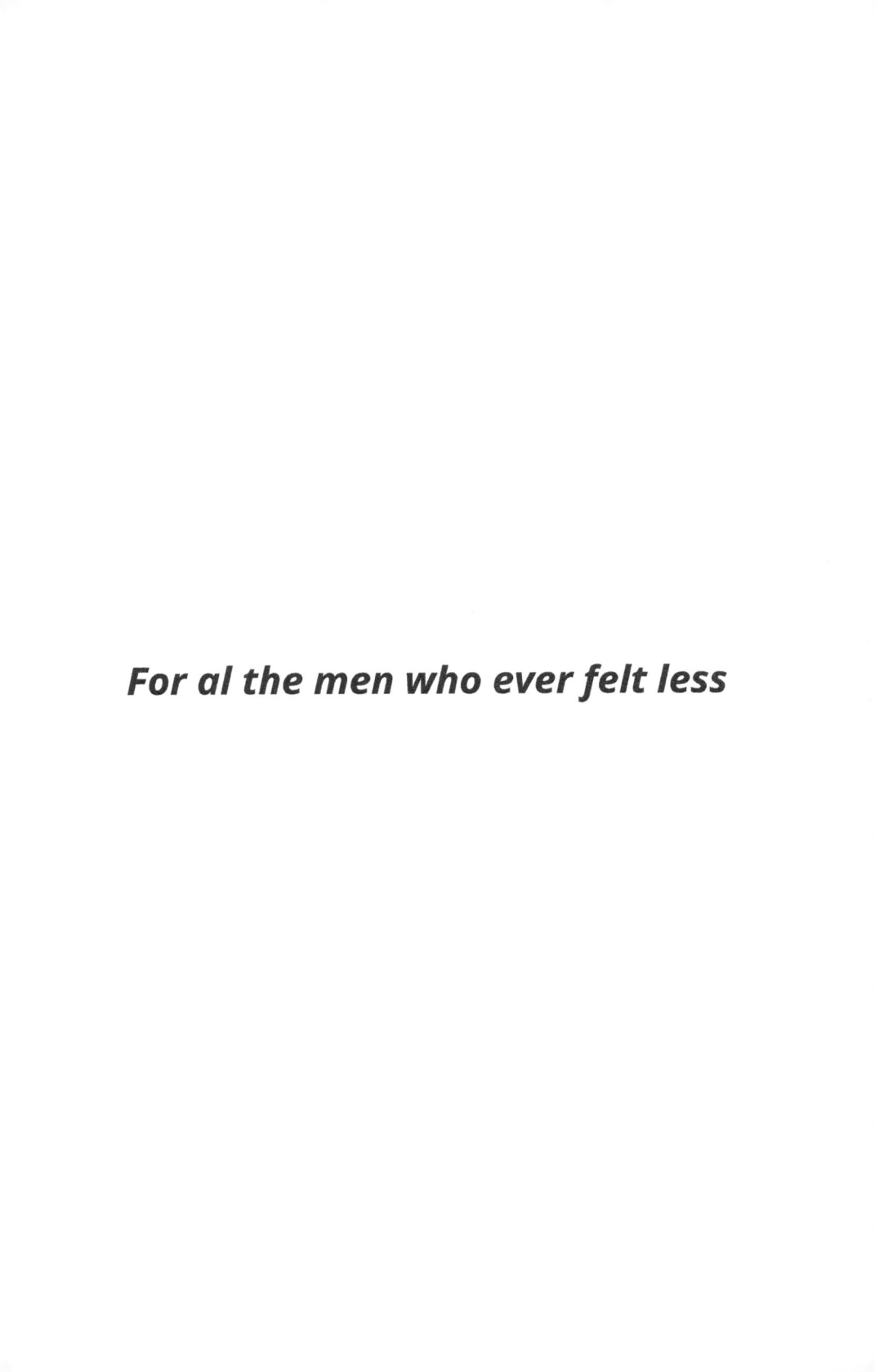

"Being a male is a matter of birth. Being a man is a matter of choice." — Edwin Louis Cole

Welcome

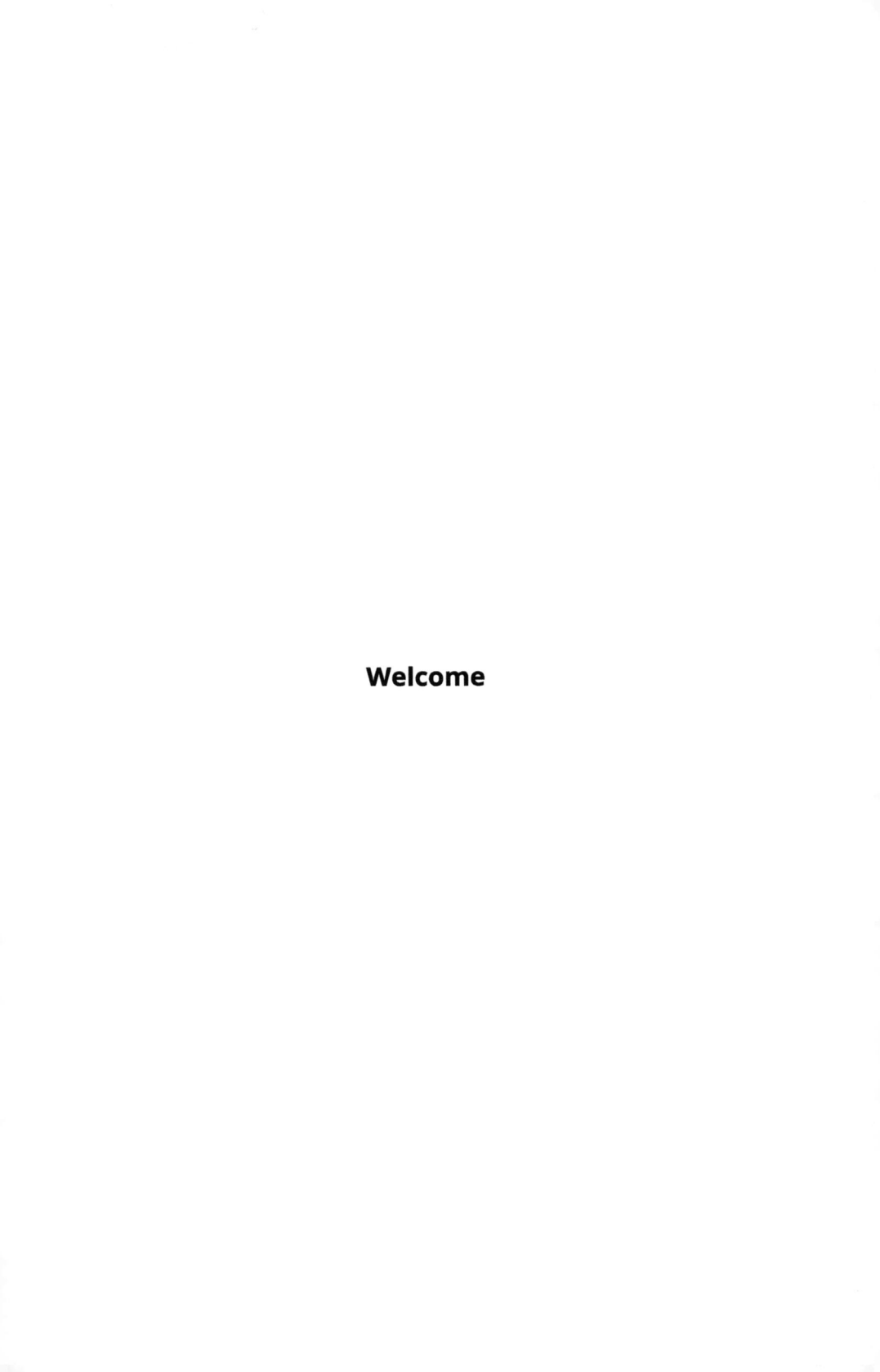

Male Body Positive

Often forgotten or not talked about, male body positivity is an important social issue facing young, middle aged and older men everyday. This book is a tool to not just be happy in your skin but to thrive an be the man you always wanted to be.

So you want to embrace who you are, that is great, this book will hopefully give you the tools to Do just that. We will learn that being male in the modern world is not as easy sit used be.

We are expected to be many things to many people. And the perfect male body is defined so closely by social media, and the community that it is hard to not be self conscious.

So much is written and said about female body positivity, it is hard to not see the endless. Articles blaming men for objectifying women, yet. Let's face it men are objectified just as much. It may not be so obvious but It is there.

We will focus on some core tips and skills that you can use to focus your energy on you, not the Noise in the background.

However, at the end of the day it is you who needs to Want to change.

Only you have that power.

"There is nothing noble being superior to your fellow man; true nobility is being superior to your former self." Winston Churchill

Step One

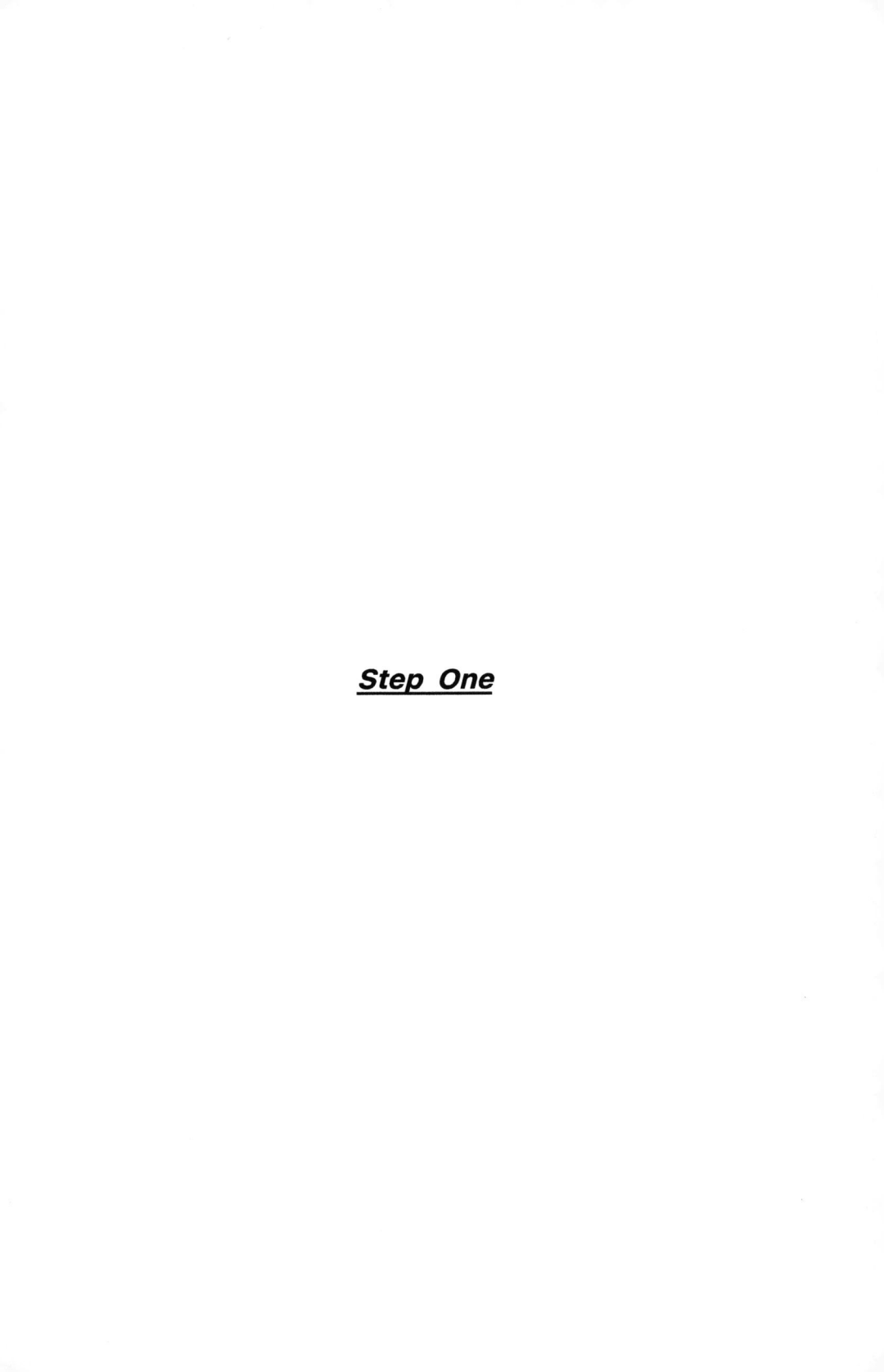

Step one, day one, task one, what ever you wish to call it, but this one is going to be the easiest for some and the hardest for others.

It is a test of your mind, and a test of your desire to improve and embrace yourself.

The male body is stunning, think for a moment about the shape, the penis, the legs, the torso, the. Balls, everything, its all magic, and it comes in so many shapes, sizes, colours, and formats.

Today, I want you to view that

beauty.

Take off your clothes, underwear too. Ideally in a private place, or at least in the locker room.

Take off everything, put your phone down, we are not taking selfies for your profiles.

Take it all off.

Now look.

FIrst thing you will look at cause we al do is your penis.

Look at it, admire the power, the veins, the Joy.

Then look at the tummy, the thighs, the arms, every inch.

Now you ma be unhappy, and that is okay, do not fee bad that you feel bad.

But I want you to look at yourself and find just one thing you love. It may be the colour of your skin, the shape of your pecs

Whatever it is admire it. Now use that image and save it in your mind forever.

You may've seen things you want to improve.

This book is not going to force you to wake up early and workout.

But if you are unhappy with your 5 kilos of christmas weight, then mate, you know what to do.

"First find the man in yourself if you will inspire manliness in others" Thomas Alcott said

Step Two

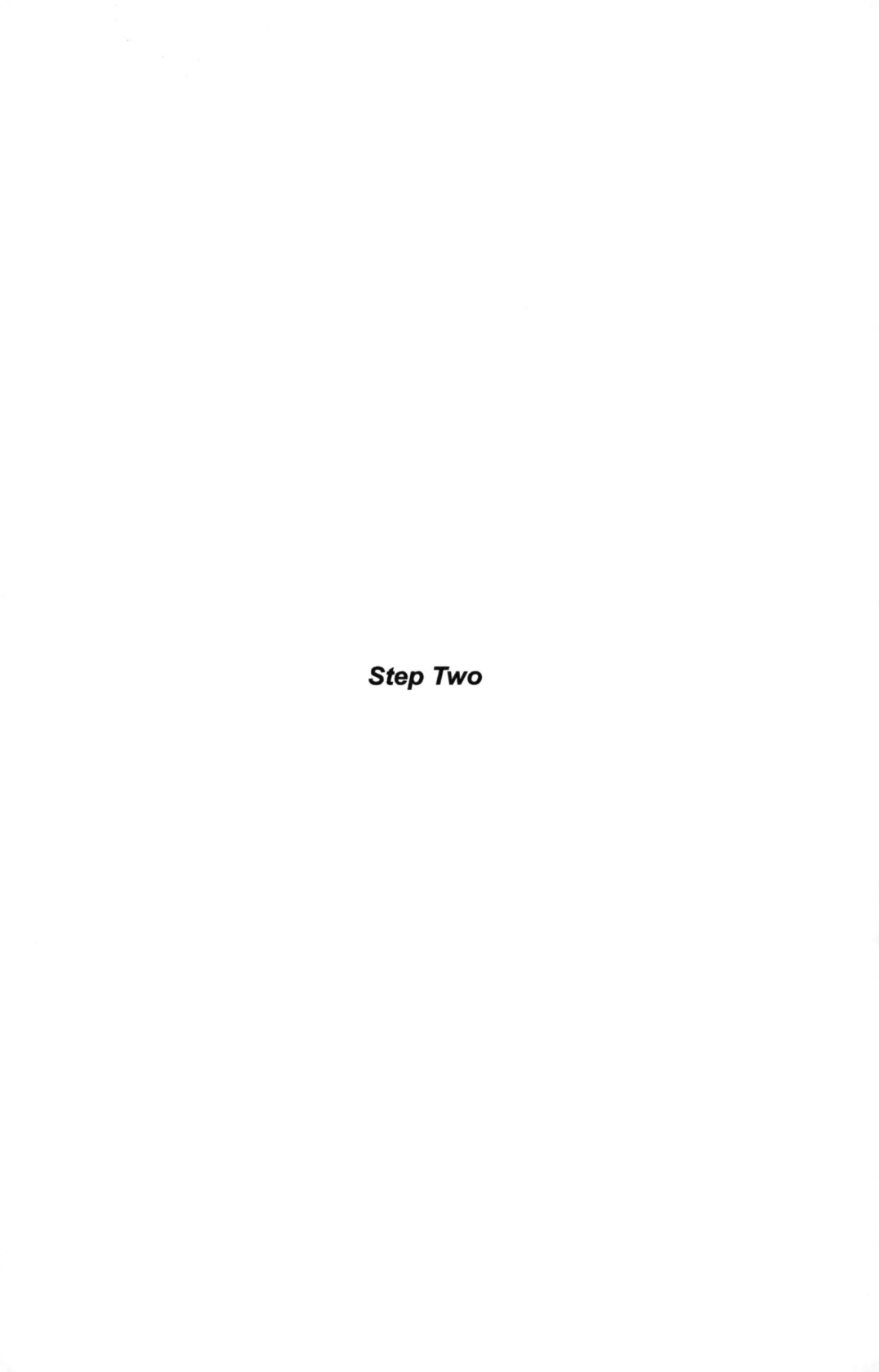

Yesterday you were naked, you enjoyed the view or at least put up with it.. I encourage you to do this every single day.

Now you ddid well and you should be proud, because you are on a path to becoming better.

Today we are not naked, but we. Will. Not have much more, I want you to go to your local pool, beach, or lake. Now if you say to me you can not swim I say fine. You can lay on the. Shoreline and enjoy the sun, rain or snow.

I want you to wear bright

speedos, red, blue, white, yellow.

The. Kind of speedos that you can not hide in.

But you say you do not have a speedo body.

What is a speedo body.

To me a speedo body is one that fits into a speedo.

I sometimes hear women say ewww men should not wear speedos.

Imagine if men said ewww women should not wear bikinis. We would be accused of al sorts of things, what I say to those women is shut the you know what up love.

Men you have a penis, and you have balls. If you are a lucky bastard you have big balls and an even bigger cock, if not that is fine, welcome to my world.

But you have them and if you put your speedos on and people stay omg you can see the outline of his dick and balls, say and?

SO get that speedo out, slide

them up your thighs, adjust and enjoy.

Wearing speedos is one of the most liberating and natural things a man can do.

You are free, you are there and you can not escape yourself.

There is a problem with obesity in the world.

I think if more men wore speedos, then they would be more in touch with their weight, they may opt to put the chocolates away and grab a pineapple.

Not saying it is bad to be fat, but by god it is good to be healthy.

If you are heavy now, that's fine, but wear your speedos anyway, and think to your self I need to get in shape, not so that these speedos fit better but so that I am around for many many more years to wear them .

I know some will say omg he is horrible how can he say you need to loose weight.

Well guess what, I did not, I said we need to all work on being healthy.

Enjoy the sun the eyes and the love that speedos allow you to show off.

If you are heavy or feel to big for them, know this.

Eveeyman in shorts on the beach is probably thinking he wishes he had the courage to do what you are doing right now. So go on you!

"I've failed over and over and over again in my life and that is why I succeed."
– Michael Jordan, athlete

Step 3

So, tell me how did the speedos feel.

Are you a new fan, or a new hater? It is okay.

If you did not like it that's fine, and that's part of life. We can not love every single moment.

Today we will do something less intimidating, less public.

Now I encourage you to do this wearing your speedos, but if you do not that's fine, I will survive.

I want you to go get some paper, old paper, new paper, what ever you can find, and something to write with.

Today I want you to write a story about your body, it can be fun, sad, erotic, meaningful, what ever.

It does not need to be an award winning book, or filled with amazing tales.

I want you to write a story. This will help you connect with yourself on a more meaningful level.

This will help you see and think about your body in a way you maybe never did before.

What ever the story is I encourage you to read it, cry over it, laugh over it but mainly to feel it.

"I'm 37 and finally love and accept myself. This isn't a 'good for me' post. And it's definitely not a 'feel bad for me post.' It's for the kids who don't take their shirt off at the pool. Have fun. You're wonderful and awesome and perfect." — *Jonah Hill*

Step 4.

How was the story, did you enjoy writing it, and more so did you enjoy reading it.

We have so many stories to tell, so many memories.

Often no one seems to listen, or maybe it is that no one has time, but what ever it is this is your story. Tell it to no one, or tell it to all. The main thing is you have heard it, you have felt it, you have lived it.

You have worked hard. You have tried to be a better man.

Sometimes just thinking about bettering yourself if the best way to becoming better. I mean think about those days you were tired and you went right mate, snap outta it you have to get to work.

Well sometimes the placebo effect is real.

So today, I want you to think of a man you would conciser to have the perfect body.

I am thinking billy Slater, a famous NRL player.

Now there is a fella who can wear speedos and make the world stop.

I want you to look at that fellas body, thee one in your mind, and I want you to think, okay, it's amazing, I could be like that too. But, I chose life, I chose food, I chose friends, I chose to sleep in.

It's okay to not be perfect you see that guy with that amazing body has his own issues, his own hang ups and his own sacarfices.

It is healthy to look at other men and aspire to be like them.

Hey its great, I know when I am tired at the gym, I just need to look at my gym buddy Travis, who has the best legs I have ever seen, and think okay one more rep.

But what is not okay is looking at our mate, that celebrity or whoever and thinking they are perfect, they may have the body you desire, but they have issues. We all do.

I have heard so many times.

If I could just drop 5.kgs before that party I will be happy.

You maybe happy for the moment when you slide your jeans on. But is that really your source of happiness, or is it a lifelong journey or memories, hard work and. happiness.

So does it take just 4 days to be a better man who is at peace with his body.

Take these tools. Work on yourself, and strutt in your speedos all summer long.

Milton Keynes UK
Ingram Content Group UK Ltd.
UKHW050436280324
440101UK00016B/1117